Eat to Perform

Boost Energy,

Sharpen Your Mind,

Live Longer

By

Odelia Rosie

Eat to Perform: Boost Energy, Sharpen Your Mind, Live Longer

Copyright © 2017

ISBN: 9781520252766

Warning and Disclaimer

Every effort has been made to make this book as accurate as possible. However, no warranty or fitness is implied. The information provided is on an "as-is" basis. The author and the publisher shall have no liability or responsibility to any person or entity with respect to any loss or damages that arise from the information in this book.

Publisher Contact

Skinny Bottle Publishing

books@skinnybottle.com

SKINNY
BOTTLE

Introduction

You are what you eat. We've heard this saying for so many times, and it's actually not that hard to understand what it means. Unfortunately, many people, probably including you, do not give much importance to what this statement means. Yes, we all know that our diet—the types of foods we put on our plate, the snacks we munch on when we're hungry, and the contents of the food stash you keep hidden in your closet, all affect our health. Yet, most people still choose to give in to their guilty pleasures, binge on junk food when they feel stressed and continue to maintain their unhealthy diet. What's the result of this? A population of unhealthy and overweight individuals.

Of course, I wouldn't be confidently bold to claim this if there aren't any medical studies and statistics to back me up.

• In 2014, the World Health Organization (WHO) reported that 39% percent of the world's adult population (1.9 billion individuals 18 years old and above) are overweight. Of this number, a staggering 600 million were reported to be obese. As we all know, being overweight or obese puts you at high risk of developing chronic diseases and can directly affect the quality of life you're living.

According to WHO, being overweight or obese is caused by an "energy imbalance between calories consumed and calories expended." Which simply means an unhealthy diet loaded with high-calorie foods, plus a sedentary lifestyle can definitely lead to overweight and obesity.

• A study published in the Federation of American Societies for Experimental Biology showed that the experimental rats who were fed a high-fat diet (a.k.a. junk foods and fast foods) for nine straight days had significantly reduced physical endurance and a decline in their cognitive ability.

• Another study also showed that consuming foods with trans-fat (a.k.a. bad fats), which are present in junk food can interfere with the brain's function in sending signals throughout the body.

• One study also showed that although a fast food meal for lunch can make you feel satiated after a long morning at work, it can actually deplete your energy levels instantly, making you feel even more tired and fatigue; which makes accomplishing tasks even harder.

Health experts also agree that a diet where all meals are empty calorie foods can lead an individual to suffer from chronic fatigue.

• Since junk food lacks the nutrients and other vitamins that your body needs, consuming it often can directly affect your mood, therefore also interfering with your productivity. In fact, scientists from the University of Granada in Spain showed that individuals who have a diet filled with fast food and commercially baked goods are 51% more likely to develop depression than those who kept a healthy diet. Another expert from the Canary Islands claimed that "Even eating small quantities is linked to a significantly higher chance of developing depression."

• An unhealthy diet filled with saturated fats and trans-fat increases the bad cholesterol in the body. Over time, the bad cholesterol will stick to the wall of the arteries which will block the flow of blood to the heart; and then can eventually lead to heart attack or other cardiac ailments. According to WHO, cardiovascular diseases (CVD) are the number one cause of death globally. In 2012, 17.5 million people died because of CVD.

Knowing how seriously we should consider our diet and how it directly affect our health and performance, I hope that by now, you're totally convinced that you need to do something to turn things around. Even if all your life you've been consuming unhealthy foods, now is the time to do what is right.

I've divided this book into five different chapters—one for the body, how you can increase your energy, strength, and stamina; second, what foods to eat to improve your mental health, which includes your memory, sharpness, and focus; third, foods that support your heart's health, to prevent cardiovascular diseases; fourth is about eating the right foods to getting quality sleep, which is vital for your overall health; and finally, foods that will increase your longevity.

Although the main focus of this book is foods and their benefits, I've also included some tips in the chapters, which can further increase your performance and promote your health.

Treat this book as your bible to guide you in choosing the right type of foods that you should include in your diet. I hope you enjoy reading!

Foods that Boosts the Body's Performance

Ever wondered why you suddenly feel out of energy and sleepy after eating a bag of chips for your afternoon snacks? That's because junk food is packed with trans-fat, calories, and sugar that can make your energy crash after eating them. Not only is your energy affected by eating junk food, even your muscles are!

Monosodium Glutamate, or what we know better as MSG, are found in fast foods and processed food. MSG is added to these foods as a flavor and color enhancer. Although MSG makes food taste and look good, it is also seen to cause the muscles to weaken; it can even cause headaches and even hormone fluctuations!

If you're looking to boost your energy, endurance, and strength, as well as improve your mobility, then it's time that you empty your cupboard (yes, even your secret stash) with junk food and processed foods and replace them with natural and healthy foods that are proven to improve the body's performance.

Here is the list of the best food choices you can stock your pantry with:

• *Sweet Potatoes*— This humble root vegetable that is often used as an alternative to the famous white potato, is rich in nutrients such as vitamin C, beta-carotene, manganese, and is a great source of dietary fiber.

According to nutritionists, when sweet potatoes are partnered with lean protein, it spurs the repairing and rebuilding of muscles, which is needed especially after heavy training. Sweet potatoes are in fact one of the popular snacks for athletes and workout enthusiasts who wish to keep their energy stores high.

- *Bananas*— A study from a university in North Carolina showed that bananas are just as effective as sports drinks when it comes to providing cyclists the energy they need during intense training. That's because bananas provide loads of potassium (a type of electrolyte) that is lost during workout sessions.

Tip: Always remember to replenish your body's electrolytes before or after working out if you want to avoid muscle cramps, spasms, and fatigue.

- *Avocados*— You may see avocados in many healthy food diets, that's because the health benefits that this fruit has is tremendous. It is rich in Vitamin C and K, B Vitamins (which are also known as "energy and stress vitamins"), dietary fiber, and healthy fat, which can be used by the body as fuel for energy.

Another good thing about the avocado is that it is a very versatile ingredient for your meals—you can enjoy its creamy goodness as a shake, in your salads, or even in your hot meals. Your creativity in the kitchen is the only thing that can limit you when you're using avocado for your recipes.

- *Grapefruit*— For people who wish not only to improve their body's energy levels but also lose weight as well, the grapefruit is one item that you need to add to your grocery list. Many studies have proven that one of the benefits of consuming this citrus fruit is to help the body lose weight. You can enjoy this benefit when you regularly consume grapefruit with your salads or as a snack, and even when you drink it as juice.

• *Raisins*— Those wrinkly bits you avoid when eating trail mix is actually a great source of carbohydrate that your body can use as energy during a workout or any strenuous activities that you're going to do. Not only that, it's also very rich in antioxidants, which helps decrease inflammation.

• *Pumpkin Seeds*— If you find yourself catching your breath during exercise, chances are, your body is lacking iron. This mineral is essential in producing red blood cells that bring oxygen throughout the body. Pumpkin seeds (and even squash seeds) are great sources of plant-based iron, which can help the efficient delivery of oxygen-rich blood to your body and also prevent fatigue.

• *Acai Berries*— Compared to the other fruits on this list, this berry is probably the least popular one. However, it is one of the healthiest in this list because it is loaded with anti-oxidants, phytonutrients (a compound found in plants proven to help prevent various illnesses), vitamins, and minerals that are beneficial for the body. Known as a superfood, the Acai berry is also seen as a great source of natural sugar to help boost your energy.

Tip: If you're having a hard time looking for fresh acai berries, you can opt to shop for dried of frozen acai, or even acai juice, and still reap the same benefits of this nutritious berry.

• *Kale*— Another superfood on this list is kale. This green leafy veg is also rich in vitamins and minerals, but is better known for its high levels of antioxidants that help increase the supply of oxygen to the blood; therefore also improving the body's stamina.

Tip: Even if you're not athletic, but want to a sudden boost of energy, adding a cup of kale in your salad or smoothie will do the trick.

• *Cottage Cheese*— Are you looking for a vegetarian-friendly source of protein for your active lifestyle? Then, cottage cheese is one of your best choices for it. Not only is it a good source of protein, but it also contains compounds that can help repair and rebuild muscles after workouts.

• *Eggs*— This breakfast staple is a great food choice to increase your body's performance because it provides the protein and micronutrients that are needed to help build and repair muscles, as well as to nourish the body.

Tip: Consume some hard-boiled or soft-boiled eggs and your choice of carbs to help balance your body's response to stress and avoid muscle breakdown during your workout sessions.

• *Ginger*— If your mobility is being affected by joint pains, then you must consider adding ginger to your stews, soups, or even your smoothies! A famous ingredient in Asian dishes, the ginger root provides loads of benefits to the body, including reducing inflammation and providing relief to join pains. Some studies even recognize ginger as having the same effects with ibuprofen.

• *Salmon*— Another good source of dietary protein is salmon that can help prevent muscle breakdown. Also, this fish, along with the other types of fishes rich in omega-3 fatty acids (like mackerel, sardines, and tuna) can decrease inflammation, which can cause sore muscles and injuries, which especially affects athletes.

- *Beef*— Preferably grass-feed beef, this meat contains loads of iron that can refill the body's lost energy after workouts. It is also rich in protein and amino acids that help the body recover from strenuous activities making this a perfect after workout meal.

- *Bone Broth*— Packed with vitamins, minerals, amino acids, and all other good nutrients, bone broth is probably one of the cheapest foods/ingredients that fight inflammation, therefore reducing your bouts with joint pains, and giving you an improved mobility.

Tip: You can easily buy ready-made bone broth in the grocery if you don't have enough time to make one for yourself. However, it will be wise if you take note of the sodium content (or added salt) of the item you're buying. If you want to keep your blood pressure in healthy levels, then you must stay away from foods that have high salt content.

- *Olive Oil*— This is obviously one of the known healthiest ingredients on the planet. But what many don't know is that adding one to two tablespoons of extra virgin olive oil to cooked meals can provide the body a good source of fat and nutrient-rich calories to keep up the energy stores in the body.

Use the items I mentioned above as ingredients for your next meals to improve your body's performance!

Foods that Sharpens the Mind and Improves Memory and Focus

Mental decline is an inevitable part of aging—this is what most people most people believe. That's why there is a term called "senior moments" when adults tend to forget things or have a hard time recalling what they're about to do or say.

However, according to health experts, although older adults will experience a certain amount of mental decline, it doesn't mean that memory loss is an inevitable part of growing old. Likewise, other mental activities such as the ability to form judgment and arguments, common sense, and the ability to do the same things as before, is not affected by normal aging.

You have to understand that no matter what age you are, whether you're a teenager, an adult, or is already in your twilight years, you still have the ability to improve your memory and focus, and even protect your gray matter. That's because until you're healthy and alive, your brain is capable of producing new brain cells and has the capability called "neuroplasticity" where it can grow and change its form as a response to its environment.

Now, the question is, why do some people experience grave memory loss? Why do they suffer from cognitive decline?

Think of your brain as a muscle, without exercise and healthy diet to keep it strong and healthy, it will grow weak and decay over time. That's why neurologists recommend for us to practice our brain every day; whether it's as simple as learning something new, solving puzzles, or calculating math problems—all these contribute to making our mind sharp and improving our memory.

Of course, our diet takes an important part in our brain's health. In fact, a study that was presented at the Society for Neuroscience meeting in 2014 reported that the diet from birth (even the mother's diet while the baby is still in the womb) until an individual grows as an adult, affects his or her brain health.

However, like I said, it's not too late to support your brain's health by keeping it active every day and choosing the right foods to eat to combat memory loss, improve your focus, and sharpen the mind.

Here is a list of the best foods to boost your brain's power:

- *Whole-Grains*— Consuming this will not only enable you keep away fat and prevent your sugar levels to spike but eating whole grains such as oatmeal, brown rice, whole-wheat pasta, and bread, can help keep your focus sharp throughout the day.

That's because, just like any other parts of our body, our brain also needs energy (in glucose form) to focus. Foods with low glycemic index, such as whole grains, releases glucose in our bodies slowly, therefore providing us with a steady flow of fuel for energy all day.

- *Fish rich in omega-3 fatty acids*— Other than being a good source of protein and preventing inflammation, omega-3 rich fishes are found to also promote heart and brain health. DHA, which is the particular omega-3 fatty acid found in fish, are seen to help lower the risk of developing dementia, particularly the Alzheimer's disease for older adults.

• *Blueberries*— They may be small in size, but blueberries are one of the healthiest snacks you can munch on because it is loaded with antioxidants that can help prevent cognitive decline. In fact, studies have identified a phytonutrient present in blueberries that not only strengthens the neurons but also help improve the brain's ability to learn and remember.

A study with older adults as participants showed that drinking at least 2 cups of blueberry juice daily in the span of three months helped significantly improve their scores on cognitive tests.

Tip: Nutritionists recommend adding at least one cup of blueberries (either fresh, frozen, or dried) to your daily diet to improve your brain health.

• *Nuts*— More reason to munch on nuts for snacks! Eating nuts, particularly almonds and walnuts, are seen to support the brain's health. That's because nuts contain Omega 3 and 6 which help boost the brain's function. In fact, a study from UCLA reported that adults who ate at least half a cup of walnuts every day have higher levels of cognitive functions than those who didn't have walnuts in their daily diet.

• *Pumpkin Seeds*— Rich in zinc, consuming pumpkin seeds help in improving our brain's function such as memorizing and thinking. According to nutritionists, all you need is to eat a handful of pumpkin seeds to achieve the recommended daily amount of zinc that our brain and body need.

Tip: One easy way to add pumpkin seeds to your diet is to crush or grind them (you can use a food processor to do this) and then sprinkle them in your soups, sauces, salads, and even smoothies!

• *Chia Seeds*— One ingredient that has been becoming even more popular in the recent years is the small, but nutrient dense, chia seeds. Also recognized as a super food, chia seeds has loads of Omega-3 fatty acids and fiber. Add a teaspoon of this to your smoothies to boost the antioxidants in your body, which is not only beneficial for the brain's health, but also for your overall wellbeing.

• *Quinoa*— This is another ingredient that you should start considering storing in your pantry. As a good alternative for rice or pasta (a gluten-free option!), quinoa is a healthy source of complex carbs as well as fiber, which both help to maintain the body's blood sugar in desirable levels and at the same time provide the vital glucose that the brain needs.

• *Tomatoes*— Another antioxidant-rich food that you want to add more to your diet are tomatoes. That's because tomatoes contain a carotenoid called lycopene that protects the brain from damages caused by free radicals which can develop into dementia. (Lycopene also helps clear bad cholesterol which makes tomatoes good for the heart too!)

• *Avocado*— Again, this creamy fruit is not only good in giving our energy a boost, but the high levels of Vitamin E found in avocados are proven to help improve our brain's function and as well as sharpen our focus and memory.

- *Broccoli*— You have to thank your mom for forcing you to eat broccoli when you were young because now you're used to eating this nutrient-dense vegetable. Broccoli is rich in calcium, iron, fiber, beta-carotene, as well as Vitamins B, C, and K, which are all helpful in preventing free radical damage. It also contains a micronutrient called choline that promotes the brain's development and help improve the brain's ability to retrieve information.

- *Spinach*— No wonder, Popeye couldn't get enough of this leafy veg— because it is one of the healthiest foods not only for our body but our brain as well. This vegetable contains lutein, a type of anti-oxidant that helps sweep toxin in the brain.

An experiment at Tufts University in Massachusetts also showed that spinach can help improve one's focus and memory. According to the study, students who regularly ate spinach had better academic performances than those who didn't have spinach in their diet.

Tip: Not actually a fan of eating green leafy vegetables? No worries! You can throw in a cup of spinach, with your favorite fruits, like blueberries in the blender so you can mask the veggie taste with the fruity goodness of the berry! This is an easy and wise way to consume your veggies if you don't love eating them.

- *Dark Chocolate*— This may surprise you, but yes, dark chocolate can help improve your alertness and keep you sharp. It also has a compound called flavonol that enhances the flow of blood in the brain, which in turn also helps improve its health. Of course, it is recommended that you stick to only one square inch every day, so don't go overboard! (Dark chocolate is also found to be good for the heart too!)

Foods that Support the Heart's Health

Maybe your purpose of downloading this book is to improve your physical strength or probably to know which types of food can help boost your memory. It's OK to be conscious about your physical fitness, as well as the sharpness of your brain, however, it's also important for you to also take care of your heart if you want to improve your overall performance and live a quality life.

As we all know, fatty, sugary, and cholesterol laden foods are all bad for our belly, but how about the heart? How can an unhealthy diet affect the heart?

Yes, foods rich in cholesterol can add rolls of fat to our body over time, but another thing that you should be concerned about is that a high cholesterol diet causes a build-up in our arteries, which can lead to a stroke or heart attack.

Foods that are high in sodium (salty foods) are linked to hypertension or having high blood pressure. When you have this condition, you have a higher risk of developing other serious heart health conditions. The Institute of Medicine recommends up to a teaspoon of table salt each day for people who don't have existing heart problems, but a little less than that is recommended for those who already have cardiac ailments.

Of course, you already know that if you really want to keep your heart healthy, then you should start filling your plate with vegetables and fruit—foods that are rich in fiber, while also restricting yourself from consuming foods that are high in "bad fats" (saturated fats and trans-fats) and salty foods. But, what exactly are the foods that can help improve our heart's health?

Here is the list of the top heart-healthy foods:

• *Old-fashioned Oats*— Because oats contain high levels of soluble fiber, it actually helps clean the digestive track by eliminating the cholesterol in it. Therefore, cholesterol will no longer be absorbed into the bloodstream, keeping your heart healthy and free of bad cholesterol.

Tip: It would be wise to stay away from instant oatmeal because they may contain added sugar that can cause your blood sugar levels to spike. Stick with the old-fashioned or quick-cooking oats instead.

• *Berries*— Strawberries, blueberries, raspberries...take your pick! Studies have found that the compound found in berries called anthocyanin, can help lower blood pressure, and even enlarge the blood vessels, decreasing your risk of developing heart attack when you include them in your daily diet.

• *Apples*— The adage "An apple a day keeps the doctor away," couldn't be more true, especially when it is about keeping your heart healthy. A research in Iowa that lasted for 20 years, found that women who were apple eaters had a lower risk of dying from coronary heart disease and other cardiovascular diseases. This is probably because of the high level of flavonoids found in apples that lowers the bad cholesterol in our body and also prevents plaque build-up in the arteries.

• *Salmon*— This probably doesn't surprise you anymore, since you already have seen salmon listed in the previous chapters as one of the best choices for a healthy body and mind. But of course, salmon and other types of fishes that contain omega-3 fatty acids can help prevent plaque build-up (therefore lowering your risk of suffering a stroke or a heart attack), decreases your risk of experiencing irregular heartbeat, and it also lowers the levels of triglycerides (fat found in the blood).

Tip: Health experts recommends consuming omega-3 rich fishes at least twice a week for a healthy heart. You can complement this by also consuming omega-3 dietary supplements.

• *Tofu*— This great source of protein, plus other soy products, like soy milk, contain loads of good fat (polyunsaturated fats), vitamins, and minerals, which all act to help reduce blood pressure. In fact, an observational study published in 2011 reported that replacing refined carbohydrates with soy products can help prevent and even treat hypertension.

• *Pinto Beans*— Like the other heart-healthy foods in this list, pinto beans, or beans in general, contain loads of soluble fiber. This help bind bad cholesterol that prevents it from being absorbed by the body. Also, there are other components in beans that can help protect the heart and keep it healthy.

Tip: Do you have high levels of cholesterol? Health experts say that consuming as little as a half cup of pinto beans a day can help lower cholesterol. How awesome is that!

• *Potatoes*— Some may tell you to avoid potatoes because they're "white" (usually, anything white in the weight loss diet world is avoided). However, dietitian Lauren Graf argues that potatoes indeed contain loads of health benefits. "They are definitely not a junk food or refined carbohydrate," Graf says, in a published article online. That's because they are rich in fiber and potassium that can help lower blood pressure and also decreases your risk of developing cardiac ailments; of course, as long as they're not cooked deep fried.

• *Olives*— Adding olives to your salads and cooking your meals with olive oil can help keep your heart healthy. That's because olives are a great source of monounsaturated fats (the good kind of fat) that lowers both cholesterol and blood sugar levels. A research published in the New England Journal for Medicine found that individuals who followed the popular Mediterranean diet (a diet with lots of veggies, fruits, grains, and of course, olives), reduced their likelihood of developing heart attacks by 30%.

• *Green Tea*— This popular drink in Asia that has also been gaining the spotlight in Western countries delivers loads of health benefits. One of which is lowering the risk of developing cardiovascular ailments (because it contains an antioxidant called catechin) when you drink four or more cups of it daily.

• *Red Wine*— Yes! Besides dark chocolate, red wine is one of your guilty pleasures that you can enjoy and still be healthy. That's because red wine contains polyphenol and resveratrol that can lower your risk of developing heart disease. However, I must warn you that you're only allowed to drink a one to two glasses of wine to enjoy its health benefits. Anything more than that can actually increase your risk of developing cardiovascular ailments.

Foods for Quality Sleep

Many people wish to be fit and healthy. They try to consume nutritious food and spend more time in the gym working out. However, what most people miss out is also allowing themselves to get quality sleep every night.

You might be wondering, "this is a book about performance, what does it have to do with sleeping?"—A lot!

According to the National Sleep Foundation, "Sleep is essential for a person's health and well-being." In fact, your mental health (mood, productivity, focus, etc.) and physical health when you're awake partly depend on the quality of sleep that you get. That's because when you're asleep, your body is working to keep your brain function healthily as well as to maintain your physical health in top shape (repairing of heart and blood vessels, maintaining a healthy balance of hormones, etc.).

Depriving yourself of sleep can bring you harm and could even lead to instant death (At least 100,000 car crashes every year is a result of drivers falling asleep.) Plus, lack of sleep may lead overeating and developing even more serious health problems.

Just how much sleep do you need every night? The National Institutes of Health suggests that adults should sleep seven and a half, up to nine hours every night for them to function at their peak during the daytime.

If every adult is required to sleep at least seven and a half hours every night, how come many don't enjoy to sleep that long? Well, there are a lot of factors such as busy schedules, stress and anxiety, and surprise, surprise—diet. Obviously, drinking caffeinated beverage can make sleeping harder for you, but also does eating large meals before going to bed (the uneasy feeling of being full when lying down).

If you're one of the 50 million Americans who don't get enough quality sleep every night, then now is the time that you add the foods in this list that can help you get quality sleep.

• *Jasmine Rice*— Other weight-loss diets will tell you to avoid consuming white rice since it has high glycemic index. However, white rice isn't actually that bad for you if you consume them in limited amounts. In fact, for the reason that it has high glycemic index, consuming white rice, particularly Jasmine rice can make you fall asleep faster.

• *Milk*— Dairy products, like milk and yogurt, are seen to help you sleep at night because it is a great source of calcium. Several studies have linked calcium deficiency to low quality of sleep.

Tip: Relive your childhood days and go drink a warm glass of milk before going to bed to sleep like a kid at night.

• *Bananas*— Not only are bananas good for your muscles, because of its rich potassium content, but this fruit is also loaded with Vitamin B6, which is needed by the body to produce melatonin, a hormone that induces sleep when triggered by darkness.

• *Chamomile Tea*— Drinking this tea is one of the most popular remedies to help people fall asleep. Studies show that Chamomile tea helps reduce anxiety, calm the nerves, and can help individuals to get quality shut-eye.

• *Passion Fruit Tea*— Another tea that you should consider sipping before going to bed is the passion fruit tea. According to an Australian study, this tea contains a type of alkaloid that "tricks" the nervous system into making you feel tired, therefore leader you into a deep slumber. It is recommended to drink this tea an hour before turning in for the day to help you get quality sleep.

• *Cherry Juice*— A study from the two universities from the US found that participants who drank cherry juice showed improvements in their symptoms of insomnia. According to the research, cherries have the capability to increase the levels of melatonin, a type of hormone that controls the body's sleeping and waking cycles.

Tip: Drink two ounces (divided) of cherry juice daily to help improve the quality of your sleep.

• *Cereals*— Yes, cereals are breakfast food. However, the National Sleep Foundation explains that eating cereals with milk can help you get excellent sleep at night simply because of the combination of carbohydrates (cereal) and calcium (milk) that all contributes to a sound slumber.

• *Honey*— The natural sugar content of honey increases the body's insulin levels slightly which allows the amino acid called tryptophan to enter then brain. Tryptophan is necessary in order for the brain to make serotonin, which is used to create the hormone, melatonin.

Tip: Add a tablespoon of honey to your chamomile tea before going to bed for a double dose of natural sleep-inducing effects.

• *Kale*— This, along with other green leafy vegetables such as spinach and lettuce are rich in calcium, which you now know is needed by the body to help you get quality shut-eye.

• *Salmon*— Like I said in the previous chapter, you will definitely see this fish included in these healthy food lists, so it'll be wise if you place it at the top of your grocery items next time you go out to shop. Salmon, along with halibut and tuna have high levels of vitamin B6, which is needed for the production of the sleep-inducing hormone called melatonin.

• *Shrimp*—This seafood and also lobster (and other types of crustaceans) is found to be a good source of tryptophan, which you know now is a natural sedative.

• *Elk*— This might surprise you, but elk meat is recognized to contain almost double the amount of tryptophan compared to turkey breast. Consuming elk along with healthy carbs will help this natural sedative travel faster to the brain, making want to go to bed.

Foods that Increases Longevity

What is the difference between the Japanese who has an average life expectancy of over 80 years old to Americans who are just close to 70 years old average life expectancy? That's right—diet!

Studies show that our diet contributes a huge part to our longevity. Besides the heart-healthy food in the previous chapter, there is a long list of foods that can help us live a longer life; some of these foods are:

• *Chilies*— A study from the Chinese Academy of Medical Sciences show that people who ate chilies or spicy food at least once a week in over four years can impressively lower their risk of dying by 10%. In addition, those who ate spicy meals three times every week have decreased their chances of dying by 15%.

Experts explain that capsaicin, the active ingredient in chilies that makes them hot, has properties that can prevent obesity, cancer, and reduce inflammation.

• *Lean Protein*—Lean cuts of meat, plus other alternative sources of good protein are found to also increase an individual's lifespan based on the study of the National Institutes of Health (NIH). In the study, the older adults who had high protein intake had an increase of 75% in their mortality.

However, before you go and jump into an all-protein diet, this study suggest that you limit your consumption of protein only to 10%-20% of the total of your daily calories.

• *Collard Greens*— This vegetable does not only protect the brain from cognitive decline, but it also has the properties to decrease an individual's mortality rate by 15%!

Tip: A cup or two of green leafy vegetables every day is all you need to increase your longevity, according to experts. Enjoy consuming these veggies by including them in your salads, smoothies, and even soups!

• *Winter Squash*— Orange vegetables like winter squash and pumpkins are rich in beta-carotene that is vital to keeping the body's immune system strong. They are also helpful in preventing cancer and keeping the heart healthy. Health experts recommend consuming at least one serving of beta-carotene rich veggies every day.

• *Whole-Grain*— Food items made with whole grain contains loads of fiber. Based on the study of NIH, individuals who have lots of dietary fiber in their meals have a lower risk of mortality. They explain that this is due to the fact that fiber can help promote good bowel movement and help regulate blood sugar levels (preventing type 2 diabetes).

- *Pistachios*— This type of nut, along with the other varieties, are seen to lower mortality rate by 20%, according to a research from Harvard University. Based on the study, consuming just a handful of nuts every day can significantly improve one's longevity, compared to those who rarely ate them. Although the reason is still unclear, this study suggests that it has to do with the vital minerals found in nut and its ability to help control blood sugar spikes.

- *Raspberries*— Berries to the rescue! A study from Spain found that consuming berries, along with other varieties of fruit for three to four times a week can decrease an individual's mortality by 30%. Berries, in particular, are high in polyphenols that help ward off degenerative diseases; therefore increasing your longevity.

However, it is advised to limit the consumption of store brought berry juices since they might contain added sugars and lack the fiber that the fresh berries provide.

- *Coconut*— Called as the "Tree of Life" in the Philippines because of the countless products and by-products that the coconut tree provides, it is also right to recognize that the fruit it bears, also aids in adding years to a person's life. Studies show that the coconut has properties that help the body produce hormones that slow down aging. It can also reduce inflammation, keep blood sugar in healthy levels, as well as strengthen the gut to keep dangerous microbes at bay.

Also, the coconut oil (which is also considered as a superfood), helps in promoting a better metabolism, supports the function of the thyroid, and cleanse the liver from harmful toxins.

Tip: You can use coconut oil as an alternative in cooking your stir-fry vegetables or as an ingredient for baked goods. You can also add it as an ingredient in your smoothies, or consume coconut oil supplements for better convenience.

• *Pomegranate*— Like berries, this fruit has antioxidant contents that help fight free radicals that cause aging. In fact, pomegranate is known as an anti-cancer food and can also help boost the brain's performance.

• Yogurt— This actually isn't a surprise, but a research from Japan has proven that consuming foods rich in probiotic, like yogurt, helps increase a person's lifestyle because it is able to reduce inflammation and promote a healthy gut.

Tip: Other good sources of pro-biotic are kimchi, miso soup, sauerkraut, tempeh, and pickles.

• *Coffee*— Before you rejoice and grab one of those fancy frappes from your favorite café, the type of coffee that is seen to increase longevity are the traditional (preferably black) coffee; and is limited to a cup a day. One study that focused on an island in Greece found that the residents who lived longest were those who drank a cup of Greek coffee every day. Experts explain that this is due to the antioxidants and polyphenols found in coffee that helps increase a person's longevity.

Have you created your all-new and healthy grocery list yet? What are that food items have you listed there? Make sure you avoid the junk food and processed food section on your next trip to the grocery!

Conclusion

Maybe for the longest time you've felt helpless and thought that there is no way out from your unhealthy diet and lifestyle. However, want I want you to understand is that you only need to take that first vital step in deciding that you want to change the way you eat and your bad habits in order to become healthy and perform better.

Yes, it's true that you are what you eat, so it's about time that you start consuming healthy foods.

My wish is that you will use the knowledge that you have gained from this book to help you in your journey to becoming a better and healthier you. There is no single food that can help you achieve your healthy goals, but consuming a variety of them in every meal can sure do miracles for your health and performance.

Boost your energy, sharpen your mind, improve your heart health, and increase your longevity with healthy foods starting today!

One last thing before you go. How awesome would it be if you shared your opinion about this book with a short review on Amazon? You read reviews yourself so why not give back a little to the community.

http://booksfor.review/eatperform

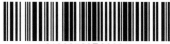

Made in the USA
Middletown, DE
15 January 2018